Yoga for Beginners:

The Ultimate Yoga Crash Course to Relieve Stress, Lose Weight, Find Inner Peace, Happiness & Heal Your Body

By Dagny Walters

Table of Contents

Copyright

responsibility of the recipient reader. Under no circumstances will any legal responsibility or blame be held against the publisher for any reparation, damages, or monetary loss due to the information herein, either directly or indirectly.

Respective authors own all copyrights not held by the publisher.

The information herein is offered for informational purposes solely, and is universal as so. The presentation of the information is without contract or any type of guarantee assurance.

The trademarks that are used are without any consent, and the publication of the trademark is without permission or backing by the trademark owner. All trademarks and brands within this book are for clarifying purposes only and are the owned by the owners themselves, not affiliated with this document.

Introduction

I want to thank you and congratulate you for purchasing this book, *Yoga for Beginners: The Ultimate Yoga Crash Course to Relieve Stress, Lose Weight, Find Inner Peace, Happiness & Heal Your Body.*

This book contains helpful information about yoga and the different ways it could benefit you. From relieving daily stress, finding your own inner peace, losing some weight, healing your body and lots more that every beginner needs to know.

This book will provide you the steps and strategies required to successfully understand and interpret the different heart rhythms!

Chapter 1: Do You Need Yoga?

Day in and day out, people experience different levels of stress, but the common denominator for everyone is finding a way to relieve it. There are many different things that one person can do but for those who are looking for something holistic, yoga would be the best option available.

Yoga is basically a set of spiritual practices and techniques which are aimed at integrating our body, mind and spirit as a means of achieving oneness with the universe. Contrary to what some people think, it is not a form of religion. Instead, it is a practice of both exploration and personal inquiry. It teaches people to be in the moment, to relish the experience of that moment and not worry about anything else beyond it.

Something that modern men and women need, considering the number of distractions and things that pull their focus away from living in the present. Unconvinced? Here are a few more reasons why you should give yoga a try:

Stress relief

Yoga is capable of reducing all the physical effects that stress has on our bodies. Because it promotes relaxation, it actually lowers the levels of cortisol. For those who are unfamiliar with it, cortisol is also referred to as a stress hormone. Too much of it can put our health at risk, so it's always best to keep it in check. Other related benefits to lowering your stress levels include: lower heart rate and blood pressure, improved digestion and a stronger immune system. Emotionally and mentally, it helps alleviate feelings of anxiety and depression along with insomnia and fatigue.

Pain relief

Yoga can also help when it comes to relieving pain. There are studies that show how practicing yoga asana along with meditation has the ability to reduce the amount of pain that people experience due to conditions such as multiple sclerosis, cancer, hypertension, arthritis, auto-immune diseases and other chronic conditions. But it doesn't end with physical pain. Yoga practitioners also compliment it for its ability to ease emotional pain.

Better breathing

Another thing that yoga teaches practitioners would be to take deeper and slower breaths. In doing this, they are actually able to improve their lung function as well as trigger the body's relaxation response, which further increases the amount of oxygen that's flowing through the body. Just think of all the benefits that more oxygen brings. For one, it helps increase focus and also aids in releasing tension that's built up in the body. Not a lot of people pay attention to it, but proper breathing is important.

Flexibility

With constant practice, it can also help improve your mobility and flexibility. The great thing about yoga is that you can work your way up the different levels, all of which have an increasing range when it comes to movements. The more you advance, the better you get and the amount of aches, and pains that you feel also significantly lessen. Just think about the fact that in the beginning, most beginners won't be able to reach their toes. But with more practice, they begin to learn how to use the right muscles and become more flexible when it comes to doing different poses.

In time, even your posture would get better and that would also help relieve pains in your back, joint, neck and shoulder muscles.

Increases Strength

The different yoga asana (poses) make use of every muscle in your body and with regular practice, you'll be able to significantly increase your strength through it. Because it also stretches muscles that are either never used or has been idle for a while, doing these poses also provides people with the additional benefit of relieving muscle tension. Something that's really great for people who work long hours and often come home with aching muscles all over their bodies. Just ten minutes of yoga could make a significant difference.

Weight Management

Despite the fact that it is much less rigorous when it comes to action, yoga can actually be used to help when it comes to weight control. It does this by reducing the cortisol levels in our bodies and burning all of the excess calories at the same time. You will be sweating and detoxifying your body the whole time you're practicing it even if you're doing the less vigorous poses, that's just fact. Besides that, it also encourages a much healthier eating habit by lowering your stress levels. This is great news for people who have a tendency to eat their emotions. With all of that combined, coupled with some discipline and a healthier diet, you should be able to reach your weight loss goals easily.

Improves Circulation

Great circulation, though often overlooked, brings about significant benefits to the body.

For one, you'll have more energy because oxygenated blood flows unhindered throughout your body and into the cells. It also helps in getting rid of the harmful free radicals in your body which often causes health issues.

Cardiovascular Conditioning

Even the gentle asana poses can provide you with pretty significant cardiovascular benefits. Among the most important would be lowering your blood pressure and heart rate. It can also help with improving your endurance as well as your oxygen uptake whenever you're exercising.

Mindfulness

Balance is important if we want to stay healthy. While we work on our body's fitness through the asana poses, yoga also takes care of our emotional and spiritual health by teaching us how to focus on the present.

It isn't uncommon for people to worry of things that have passed as well as situations that have yet to happen. All of that, piled on top of each other, shoots our stress levels through the roof. But if we become more mindful and learn how to live in the present, our worries become smaller. It also helps improve our concentration, reaction time, coordination as well as our memory.

Inner peace

Because of its meditative aspects, yoga is capable of helping practitioners with reaching a deeper, more satisfying and more spiritual place in their lives. There are people who actually practice it for this very purpose and soon found it to be an essential part of their daily living. After all, with all the chaos of life that we face every single day, carrying peace within us becomes all the more significant. It can easily affect many other areas of our lives and should we really immerse ourselves in it, it can greatly improve the quality of our day to day.

Chapter 2: Using Yoga for Weight Loss

Alright, we've already established the fact that if practiced regularly, yoga can become an effective weight loss regimen. In this chapter, we'll delve deeper into the why this is so and which yoga asana is the most effective for this purpose.

How does it help?

If you use yoga as a means of losing weight, there are many different factors that influence the process itself. The first of which would be the asana that you'll be using. These would work and stimulate all of the sluggish glands in your body, normalizing their hormonal secretions. These glands end up sluggish due to the lack of regular exercise coupled with a bad diet. The thyroid gland, in particular, has a significant effect on your weight because it directly affects the metabolism.

If you can stimulate this, your metabolic rate would increase and most of your extra fat would be turned into energy and muscle.

Another contributing factor would be the deep breathing exercises that you will be learning through yoga. In doing these exercises, you're actually increasing the oxygen intake to the cells in your body- fat cells included. What this does is boost the rate of oxidation and you end up burning even more fat. In fact, the more you do these breathing exercises, the more fat you'll be able to burn. Quite a simple and non-tedious way of losing weight, isn't it? It doesn't end there, however.

Yoga also teaches us to become mindful eaters. Most of the time, we just rush through our food without giving it much thought. This is especially so if we're under nervous strain.

We eat and eat without gaining much satisfaction hence we end up eating a lot more than we ought to. Becoming a mindful eater would change all of that. If we're able to fully appreciate a meal, we would be less frantic and enjoy it more.

Lastly, becoming a mindful eater also applies to restraining ourselves from indulging whilst in the midst of the diet. This is one of the most difficult things to do when you're on a diet. But because you'll become more aware of what it does to your body, you will develop some discipline and control towards food.

Now that we have that covered, here are some of the most effective yoga asanas that you can try for weight loss:

Ardha Chandraasana (Half-moon pose)

This pose works great when it comes to toning

the upper and inner thighs as well as the buttocks. Because it stretches the sides of the tummy, you can expect to see some fat burn in these areas too- specifically the love handles that you might have there. Lastly, it can also help with strengthening your core.

Do avoid this pose if you currently have: a spine injury, a digestive disorder and high blood pressure.

To do it: Begin by standing with your feet together. Slowly, raise both your hands above your head whilst your palms are clasped together. Extend your stretch as far as you can but do it gently. Breathe in and out slowly as you begin to bend sideways, starting from your hips. Keep your hands together. Do not bend forward and make sure that your elbows remain straight. By now, you should begin to feel a stretch going from your fingertips to your thighs. Inhale and exhale deeply as you return to the first position.

Repeat the same steps but do it with the other side of your body.

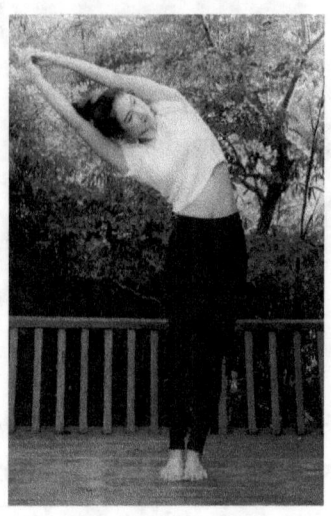

Veerbhadrasana (Warrior pose)

This asana helps with stretching your back as well as strengthening your tummy, buttocks and thighs. Do avoid this pose if you have any shoulder, back and knee troubles. People with high blood pressure should talk to their physician first or perform the pose with the guidance of a trained yoga instructor.

To do it: Begin with both your feet together, hands placed by your side. Extend your right leg slowly forward whilst you keep the other leg extended backwards. Bend your right knee forward, adjusting into the lunge position. Gently twist your torso, turning to face your bent right leg. Next, carefully turn your left food sideways to about 40 to 60 degrees, depending on your preference. Doing this should provide you with extra support. Make sure you're breathing in and out slowly as you straighten your arms, raising your away from your bent knee. Continue stretching your arms upwards while you slowly move your torso backwards. In doing this, your back should form an arch.

To return to your original position, inhale and exhale deeply while you straighten your right knee. Push off of your right leg and adjust into your original pose. Remember, don't rush any of the steps as you might end up injuring your back or your legs.

Repeat the same poses for your left leg.

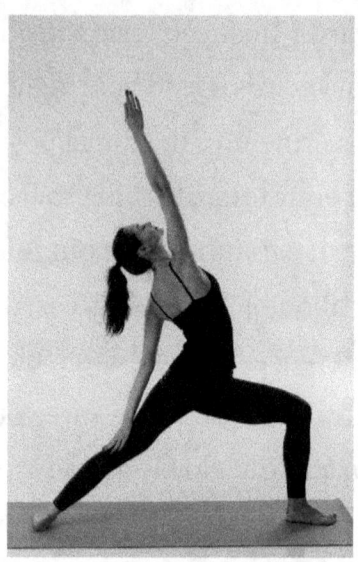

Utkatasana (Chair pose)

This strengthens the thighs and core muscles
while toning the buttocks. However, if you
have any back or knee injury, do avoid doing
this pose.

To do it: Prepare a yoga mat and stand
straight upon it, your hands in the namaste

position in front of you. Slowly begin raising your hands right above your head while you bend at the knee, making sure that your thighs are at a position that's parallel to the floor. Gently bend your torso forward just slightly while you slowly breathe in and out. Hold this position for as long as you're comfortable and once done, carefully slip back into the standing position.

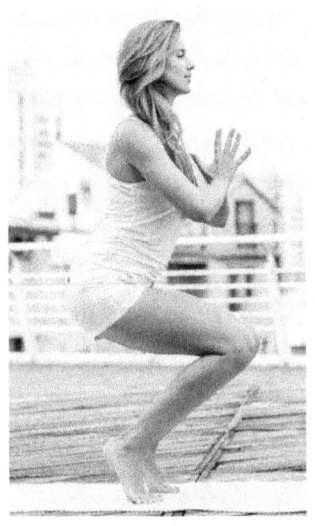

Vrkasana (Tree pose)

This particular asana is great for building your abdomen muscles as well as toning both your arms and thighs. If you have knee or back injuries, you'll still be able to do this but make sure you're being guided by a yoga instructor.

To do it: Begin by standing with both of your legs together whilst slowly shifting most of your weight over to the right one. Raise the leg that has the least amount of weight on it, make sure that your foot faces inwards when you do this, then rest it against the opposite knee. For support, you can also hold up your ankle while you're in this position.

Adjust the heel of your foot so that it now rests on your other leg's inner thigh, try to move it as close to the pelvis as possible. Once you're stable enough, raise your hands above your head and point your fingers towards the ceiling. Breathe in and out slowly and try to clear your mind even while you're maintaining your balance.

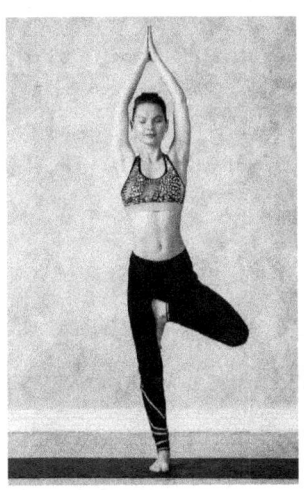

Uttansana (Forward bending pose)

This stretches the hamstrings and places some pressure on the abdomen, effectively toning it. It also has a relaxing effect on the body, given that it makes the blood rush to your head thereby making the body switch from sympathetic to parasympathetic nervous system.

To do it: Begin by standing straight and raising your hands above your head whilst you inhale slowly. After, gently bend forward and push your buttocks back until your palms are touching the floor, and your forehead is against your knees. Slowly straighten up again and repeat as much as you want.

So there you have it, just a few yoga asanas that you can interchange and use as a gentler weight loss regimen. Do make sure that you spare at least half an hour each day for practicing these as only with regular use will you see any real change.

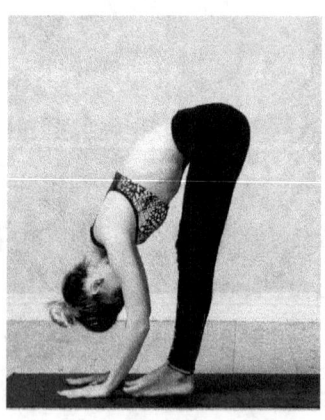

Chapter 3: Healing the Body through Yoga

There is a reason why people feel completely revitalized after doing yoga and it goes beyond clearing one's thoughts. Did you know that yoga's mind-quieting methods also have the potential to heal the body when it comes to the things that might be ailing it? There have been plenty of studies that prove how these mind and body practices stimulate healing in the body and yoga, in particular, is one of the most effective out of the lot.

Here are a few of the problems that yoga can help with fixing:

Back pain

People who have practiced yoga on a daily basis for at least a month (or more) have noted that it helped with reducing the back pain by at two-thirds. This also led to them using less and less of their pain medication.

How does it work?

Well, it has been suggested that the act of pressing down onto the floor actually activates the body's pressure receptors which then block the neural pathways where pain signals pass through. To make it work, however, it is best to skip the more rigorous yoga practices and opt for more stretching as well as meditation. The calmer and more relaxed your nervous system is, the better.

Migraines

Doing yoga every single day is known to lessen the intensity and frequency of migraines, many studies have shown. This happens because yoga helps with reducing the cortisol levels in the body hence bringing it into a state of relaxation. Stress and anxiety are two of the major causes for migraine so steering clear of those already helps in a significant way. Doing yoga also promotes easier and better sleep.

If you get ample amounts of sleep, your brain secretes far less

pain chemicals than it normally would. For this, always pick a more calming form of yoga. Something that works with proper breathing helps a lot too.

Muscle injury

Muscle injuries can range from being quite mild to something really serious which could have long term effects if left untreated. As for the reasons why it happens, this could vary greatly. To get things back in order, some rehabilitation would be needed. Doing yoga helps because each time you move and adjust your body into a particular pose, deep stretching happens and this opens the muscles up. Whenever this happens, there's an increase of oxygenated blood flow into that area and detoxification occurs. Both things help boost the recovery and healing process while strengthening the musculature at the same time.

For this, poses with just enough stretch would be perfect. Do get some advice from a professional yoga trainer since you need to make sure that the poses wouldn't further the extent of your muscle injury.

Colds and blocked sinuses

When it comes to colds, everything comes down to getting rid of stress yet again. After all, stress can significantly weakens our immune system and when that happens all sorts of illnesses enter the picture. Colds are the easiest to catch and in some cases, also quite hard to get rid of. For this, you will need to perform some restorative and calming poses. Some breathing exercises would be great too in order to help open up the nasal passageways and get more oxygen into your blood. Giving the mind a break also helps and because it boosts your immune system, you're basically providing your body with the support it needs in order for it to heal itself.

Ankle problems

Ankle sprains aren't uncommon and even a slight misstep can lead to it. If you intend on using yoga to help speed up the healing process, you would need to keep moderation in mind. You will need to recuperate first and apply ice to the injured area daily. If need be, follow your doctor's instructions before diving headfirst into doing yoga. A professional yoga instructor would be able to let you know when to begin your asanas. For this, gentle stretches would be the most appropriate as long as they don't place too much tension on your ankle.

Remember, knowledge and moderation are the keys to using yoga as a way of healing your body. If you're unsure, always ask a professional instructor. They would know which asanas would be most beneficial to your needs and just how much of it you can actually do.

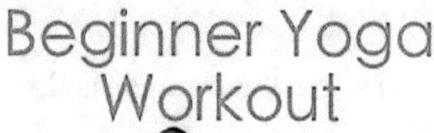

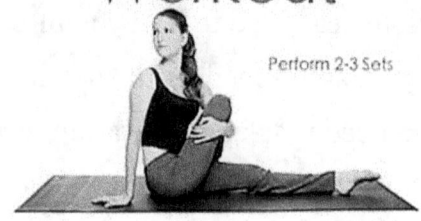

Perform 2-3 Sets

8-10 Sec. Spinal Twist

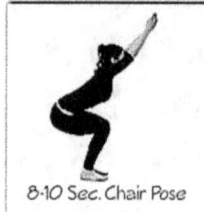

8-10 Sec. Chair Pose

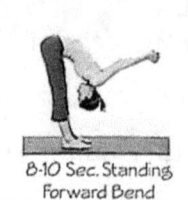

8-10 Sec. Standing Forward Bend

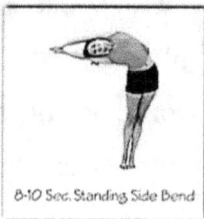

8-10 Sec. Standing Side Bend

Chapter 4: Finding Inner Peace & Happiness through Yoga

For many people, stress has become something that they simply accept as part of their daily lives. Whilst to some extent, stress can benefit us by motivating our body, mind and spirit when it comes to completing tasks and overcoming challenges. However, too much of it can eventually diminish our happiness as well as peace of mind.

Stress can be looked at on two different levels. The first of which would be the micro level and this covers all of the individual stress we face on a daily basis within the environment we move in. Then there's the macro level which covers all the stress coming from a larger scale; global issues, the economy, illnesses and society in general. You may not spare these things much thought, but as they pile on top of each other, all of them begin impeding our daily way of functioning. If we're not careful, it can result to a burn out and grind everything to a halt.

So what do we do? Well, the best solution is to start working on developing inner peace. This is basically the state of being spiritually and mentally at peace even in the face of challengers, stress and discord. It's easy to feel at ease when not much is happening in our lives but once everything takes a turn, how will we react?

Yoga teaches us meditation and how we can develop a connection with our body, mind and spirit. It enables us to let go of the worries and any excesses of the day so that we can focus internally, and on the things that truly matter. Mindfulness is another lesson that we can take away from yoga, to live in the present and not in the past or the future.

In doing so, we reduce the amount of worry and fear that we have. We can avoid being anxious for what hasn't yet passed so that we are able to focus all of our energy into working on the present, and making it the best it can possibly be.

Using yoga to achieve inner peace would help liberate our mind, body and spirit from everything that's been weighing it down. In giving ourselves these quiet moments at the start and end of each day would help detoxify us from within and provide us with much needed clarity.

There are many different types of yoga practices that you could use for this. The most popular ones are: Hatha yoga, Raja yoga, Karma yoga, Jnana yoga, Bhakti yoga, Kundalini yoga and Mantra yoga among others.

Basic Meditation for Inner Peace

- Start off by seating in the "Peace Position". This is basically where you have your legs crossed, right leg over your left one with your hands following suit. Have your palms up and your right index finger should be touching your left thumb. Rest your hands on top of your lap

- comfortably, straighten your back and breathe naturally. Close your eyes.

- Take slow and deep breaths while you relax every muscle in your body. Let your shoulders lose the tension knotted up in them, shake your hands and arms gently if needed. This is the time when you need to begin clearing your head. Imagine every worry you have slowly leaving your body as you exhale. If you have to, repeat a mantra that encourages you and makes you feel better. Repeat it in your head or speak it quietly.

If at any point, you feel distracted or if you feel as if certain parts of your body are becoming tense again, simply pause and center yourself once more.

- For beginners, keeping the mind still can be a little tricky but don't fret! This is normal and in time, with constant practice, you'll be able to have better control over your thoughts. What you need to do now is to learn how to acknowledge the presence of these unwanted thoughts but to never dwell on them. Become a passive observer instead of acting upon every emotion and every trigger. Let the experiences occur but stay neutral. Now, if you start feeling tense once more, take another deep breath and repeat your mantra as you let the thoughts pass you by. Just keep being passive and remain relaxed.

- End your meditation with a few minutes of simply breathing in and out.

Sharing the Love

In meditation, you are also taught to expand the good feeling you have after meditating. By doing so, you are also able to increase your happiness. This sharing can be done every day before and after your daily meditation. It can also help improve the quality of the meditation itself.

Aside from this, you'll also radiate a sense of happiness all the time. It doesn't matter if you're awake or asleep. A lot of yoga practitioners who do this attest to the fact that it has also given them great and meaningful dreams. If they've been experiencing grief and anger, these things begin to diminish.

Here's how you can practice it for yourself

Just before you end or start your meditation, take a few minutes to focus your mind towards the center of your body. This is the area where you feel love. Imagine that love building and turning into a bright sphere of light, add onto it by recalling all the good things that you have in your life right now. As it expands, visualize it spreading in all directions. From your body to the outside. Send your good wishes and thoughts to everyone as you do this. You may even speak your wishes out loud if this works better for you.

Chapter 5: Meditation Tips for Beginners

If you're just starting out with meditation, even the smallest things can help when it comes to enhancing the quality of your sessions. Luckily, there are many simple steps that you can take when it comes to making the experience even better. Shall we enumerate?

Mind your posture

Whether you're sitting or standing, always make sure that your spine is straight and that you're always holding your chin up. If you have bad posture, your mind has a tendency to drift more and your energy levels might go down. Remember that your mind and body are intertwined. So if your body is well-balanced, your mind would follow suit.

Count your breath

One of the biggest challenges that any beginner could encounter when meditating would be remaining focused. For this, counting your breath is an effective practice. When you breathe out, quietly count one to four then round back to one. Consider "one" your home number and going back to it is akin to returning your focus to the present

Handling your emotions

If you've been experiencing extreme emotions such as anger and grief, meditation can become quite difficult to begin. This is because your mind is in a chaotic state and would need a while before it can settle down. Expect to feel these emotions in your body once you've sat down to begin your session. You might feel a trembling in your arms and around your chest.

Your shoulders might tense up and you might feel something weird in your gut. Don't worry because all of these things are normal. Even more advanced practitioners experience them as well. Just take a few deep breaths and allow yourself some time to calm down. Your body will eventually enter a state of relaxation.

Creating your space

Lastly, do pay some attention to the area wherein you'll be doing your meditation. The more calm and cozy it is, the better it would be for your sessions. Some people prefer decorating the space wherein they meditate, adding ambient lighting and some incense to help them go into a deeper meditative state. You don't really need a lot when practicing yoga.

A simple yoga mat and a pillow to support your back would be enough.

However, you can also have some soft music playing while you go through the different asana.

For some people, the music helps prevent their mind from wandering.

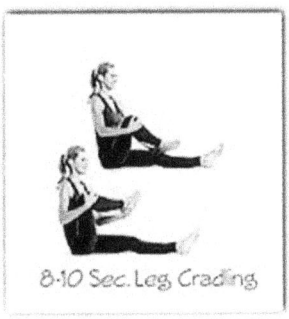

8·10 Sec. Leg Cradling

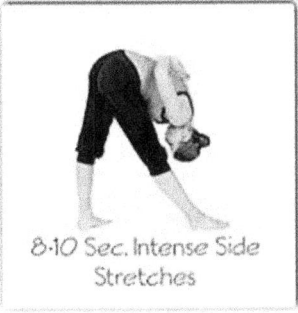

8·10 Sec. Intense Side Stretches

Conclusion

Thank you again for purchasing this book! I hope this book was able to help you learn more about Yoga for Beginners. The next step is to put this information to use, try yoga for yourself and learn about the different ways it can change your lifestyle as well as your way of thinking.